Abdominal Fat

Ways To Reduce It ·

Table of Contents

These are some of my other books below, and my website is
www.LosingBellyFatMission.com :

https://www.amazon.com/dp/B06XB4WHZX
http://www.amazon.com/dp/B06X9LXBB8
http://www.amazon.com/dp/B06WLK7497

http://www.amazon.com/dp/B06W54JKQN
http://www.amazon.com/dp/B06X6DJ9K3
http://www.amazon.com/dp/B06WGNJ9N3
http://www.amazon.com/dp/B06W549TBD
http://www.amazon.com/dp/B06VTF5DQJ
http://www.amazon.com/dp/B06WRPSBKK
http://www.amazon.com/dp/B06WD194JR
http://www.amazon.com/dp/B06WCZTK7Y
http://www.amazon.com/dp/B06X3QN1HT
http://www.amazon.com/dp/B01N19WBF2
http://www.amazon.com/dp/B01N2AVECA
http://www.amazon.com/dp/B01N4VZIAV
http://www.amazon.com/dp/B00QJJFS1C
http://www.amazon.com/dp/B01EMNO2MW
http://www.amazon.com/dp/B00SSFWCPA
http://www.amazon.com/dp/1520531230
http://www.amazon.com/dp/B01N4V7SR9
http://www.amazon.com/dp/B00SX58DUI
http://www.amazon.com/dp/B010K7YP62

http://www.amazon.com/dp/B012LAYNNQ
http://www.amazon.com/dp/B00RVX3KY2
http://www.amazon.com/dp/B01MR6SWGW
http://www.amazon.com/dp/B00XF6G4HO
http://www.amazon.com/dp/B01F1472N2
http://www.amazon.com/dp/B00PQ0TUPU
http://www.amazon.com/dp/B00PP8OZJ4
http://www.amazon.com/dp/B00QH7DY4Y
http://www.amazon.com/dp/B01052010G
http://www.amazon.com/dp/B00QDHXN7Q
http://www.amazon.com/dp/B00PO0IQIO

Among others.

Cardio Fitness For Immediate Six Pack Abs

BREATH	HIP ROLL	NORMAL	BRIDGING
10 Deep Breaths	2 Sets of 10 slow rolls each side - with 20 seconds rest	2 Sets of 10 lifts with 20 seconds rest	1 Set of 10 slow lifts. Hold for 3-5 seconds in upward phase
STANDING ROTATION	HANDS VIA KNEES	SEATED KNEE TUCKS	SUPERMANS
Alternate sides for 30 - 45 seconds	2 Sets of 10 lifts with 20 seconds rest between sets	2 Sets of 6 - 10 lifts with 20 seconds rest between sets	Alternate sides for 45 - 60 seconds

Cardio workouts and ab workouts do go hand in hand. The need to work on the abs has become very popular. Folks who are poised to burn their belly fat and getting flat abs must be ready for the challenge. The traditional cardio to the average person consists of walking on a treadmill, riding a stationary bike, work on an elliptical machine and usually watch mounted television while doing so. It takes time to get ab results by losing fat and most think that these cardio exercises will help them get rid of the fat. Hand in hand with cardio weight exercises used in bodybuilding, plus sprinting and running are great for losing flabby gut fat.

Combining lifting and sprinting alongside abs exercises will make you lose fat fast in the gut area and start to loosen fat. Stomach exercises with heart pounding cardio exercises will be great toning up the loose areas of your belly. Try to get into exercises that leave your chest heaving and sweat running off you. Try 5 minutes of lifting just beyond your comfort level, so if your usually lifting a fifty lbs, up that to 70 or 80 pounds. Do some sprints in place followed by some squats for a few minutes.

Your "cardio" will soar and you'll start to see results in a shorter amount of time. So combine your abs exercises with a fair amount of weight training and cardio exercises in your routines. Alongside this, build up to some endurance and strength training. Thus move away from the stationary bikes and treadmills. Sprinting and lifting with focused intensity and little rest breaks can condition a lot of muscles in a very short amount of time.

Some of the exercises that will give good abs are more challenging than most of the exercises you see people do in gyms. Some trainers likes to push the body to its limits to achieve a faster fat burning rate than you could have normally expected. So if you have a trainer good, the pace he chooses to help lean your body out will be determined by the different type of exercises he will have you do, the different combination of exercises and the frequency.

For Healthy Fat Stomach Exercise

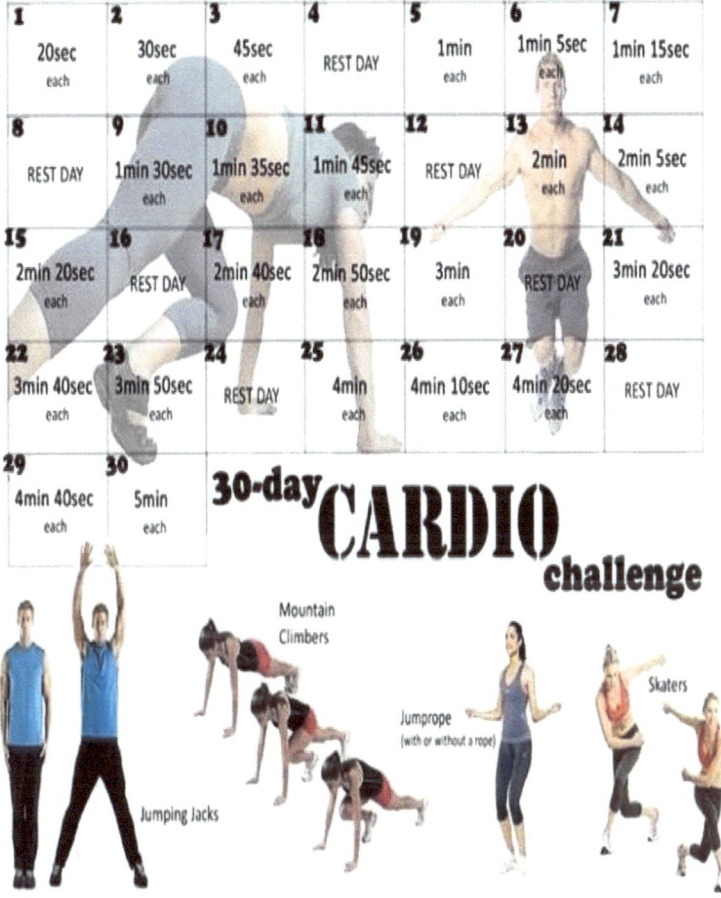

1 20sec each	2 30sec each	3 45sec each	4 REST DAY	5 1min each	6 1min 5sec each	7 1min 15sec each
8 REST DAY	9 1min 30sec each	10 1min 35sec each	11 1min 45sec each	12 REST DAY	13 2min each	14 2min 5sec each
15 2min 20sec each	16 REST DAY	17 2min 40sec each	18 2min 50sec each	19 3min each	20 REST DAY	21 3min 20sec each
22 3min 40sec each	23 3min 50sec each	24 REST DAY	25 4min each	26 4min 10sec each	27 4min 20sec each	28 REST DAY
29 4min 40sec each	30 5min each					

30-day CARDIO challenge

Jumping Jacks

Mountain Climbers

Jumprope
(with or without a rope)

Skaters

Questions on how to have a great stomach exercise are being asked a lot by people who are not satisfied with their current physique. Numerous stomach exercises are covered in abs workout. Exercises such as sit-ups, crunches, leg lifts and even the "bicycle" maneuver are great techniques to having muscle abs. But fat loss cannot be so easily achieved by just simple exercises. The maintenance of proper diet, good calorie-burning cardio exercises and a lower ab muscle toning by reverse crunches can essentially improve the state of your abdomen.

Elimination of your lower stomach fat has specific exercise techniques that you should follow religiously. The top priorities into achieving this is to eat healthy food, cardio exercises and a good night's rest are essentially the most overlooked and underestimated facts into gaining a gorgeous physique. Everyone have a difference in body fitness. There are some born skinny yet they have a bulge in the lower stomach area. Facts such as these can be frustrating as it is due to the result of our genes inside our body. Probably the most efficient in fat-burning stomach exercises are jogging and other cardio exercises such as walking or swimming.

The regular application of crunches and other stomach exercises can boost your self confidence and also increase your abdominal muscles. It is dutifully necessary for you to be working out your entire body into a sweat whilst preserving that healthy eating habit you have already started. These techniques are very important if you want to lose that stomach fat. Accomplishing a physical task such as having a firm stomach is not easy at all, but the end result is definitely worth the sweaty rigorous exercises. It is best that you should concentrate on doing your daily routine of exercise including crunches and working out with those special stomach exercise equipment in your fitness center.

It is best that you actually contribute to losing that stomach fat not just by physical exercise but also through proper diet discipline. Although any type of activity can also help in reducing that dreaded stomach fat. Start your daily routine by having a timed walk and/or jog 3-4 times a week to increase your heart's pumping strength and to also boost your body's metabolism. By increasing the rate of your metabolism, you help your body burn excess calories while you are performing your routine. Sweating is a good thing as it is your body's process of excreting toxins from your body which helps in your overall fitness. Cardio exercises such as swimming and dancing are also preferred as it is also fun exercise while working out.

Simple Cardio Exercises on a Low Budget

Stability Ball Workout

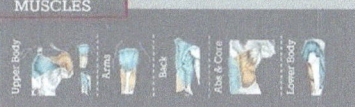

Upper Body | Arms | Back | Abs & Core | Lower Body

PERFORM WORKOUT AS FOLLOWS:
1. Select 1-2 exercises per body parts.
2. Perform the rep and set range suggested below.

Bodyweight Exercises	12-15 reps	1-3 reps
Free Weight Exercises	8-12 reps	2-4 reps

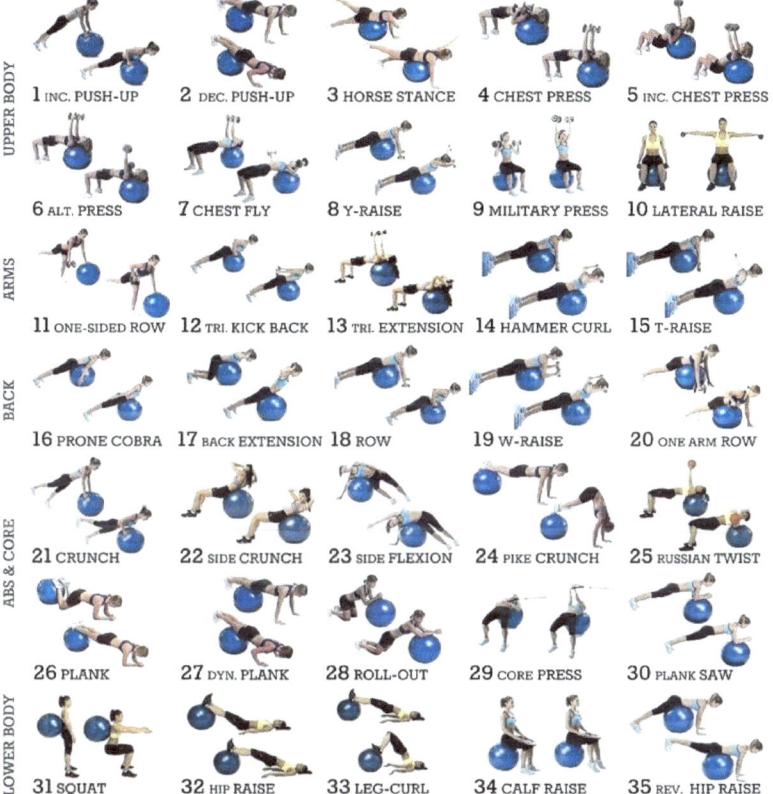

UPPER BODY

1 INC. PUSH-UP   2 DEC. PUSH-UP   3 HORSE STANCE   4 CHEST PRESS   5 INC. CHEST PRESS

6 ALT. PRESS   7 CHEST FLY   8 Y-RAISE   9 MILITARY PRESS   10 LATERAL RAISE

ARMS

11 ONE-SIDED ROW   12 TRI. KICK BACK   13 TRI. EXTENSION   14 HAMMER CURL   15 T-RAISE

BACK

16 PRONE COBRA   17 BACK EXTENSION   18 ROW   19 W-RAISE   20 ONE ARM ROW

ABS & CORE

21 CRUNCH   22 SIDE CRUNCH   23 SIDE FLEXION   24 PIKE CRUNCH   25 RUSSIAN TWIST

26 PLANK   27 DYN. PLANK   28 ROLL-OUT   29 CORE PRESS   30 PLANK SAW

LOWER BODY

31 SQUAT   32 HIP RAISE   33 LEG-CURL   34 CALF RAISE   35 REV. HIP RAISE

REPS	10-15	2-4
SETS	REPETITIONS	SETS

Most of time, overweight people are the same individuals who have low self-esteem as well as low self-confidence. This is the reason why there are so many gyms in bigger cities and towns and why every gym has its own professional gym instructors who profit financially and emotionally from assisting and helping customers lose weight the right way. Because their role is mostly a motivational one that helps us reach our goals physically and psychologically. And for those can pay the fees, it's a win-win for everyone involved. However, there are many people who cannot afford such a program. This can be a financial obstacle depending on the club or it can be more of a time obstacle because we cannot afford the time it takes to get to the gym in the nearest city center. Nevertheless, achieving our psychological and health goals does not require a gym or the outlay of cash. In fact, there are simple cardio exercises that we can do at home and at the same time we can get our dream weight after a specific period of time... and this will yield the same positive results we would expect from a personal trainer.

We all know that running is a type of exercise that is very popular and also very common; drive through any subdivision on a decent, sunny day and count the joggers running by. But running is very hard or difficult to start with if you are overweight and not even recommended if you are obese given the stress on your body. Instead of running, you should take up walking. Since you need to give a lot of energy to walking your body will be accustomed into having your heart rate go up, an essential first step to burning fat. Another simple cardio exercise is using a treadmill. If you don't want to go out and you need a lower-impact workout, then using a treadmill is best. You can always start with a lower-cost machine that will let you "graduate" to a slow running or jogging pace from a good, healthy walking pace.

Another great advantage of using a treadmill is that many of them are quiet and can be operated while watching television or while the kids or other people are asleep or need quiet. Aside from using the treadmill, you may can also get some exercise-specific DVDs like the P90X program. These are available virtually everywhere. This is also a simple and easy way to get you cardio exercise done right at home in the comfort of your living room, bedroom or other private area and generally they do not cost all that much either. And since it is a DVD, the programmers make sure there are a lot of different exercises that will provide you with enough variety to keep you engaged. Doing your simple cardio exercises at home will help you lose weight and save a few dollars and time in the process. However, if think that you need the supervision of a professional trainer, then there are in-home trainers who can come to you... but be prepared to spend a few bucks.

Four Tips For Flat Abs

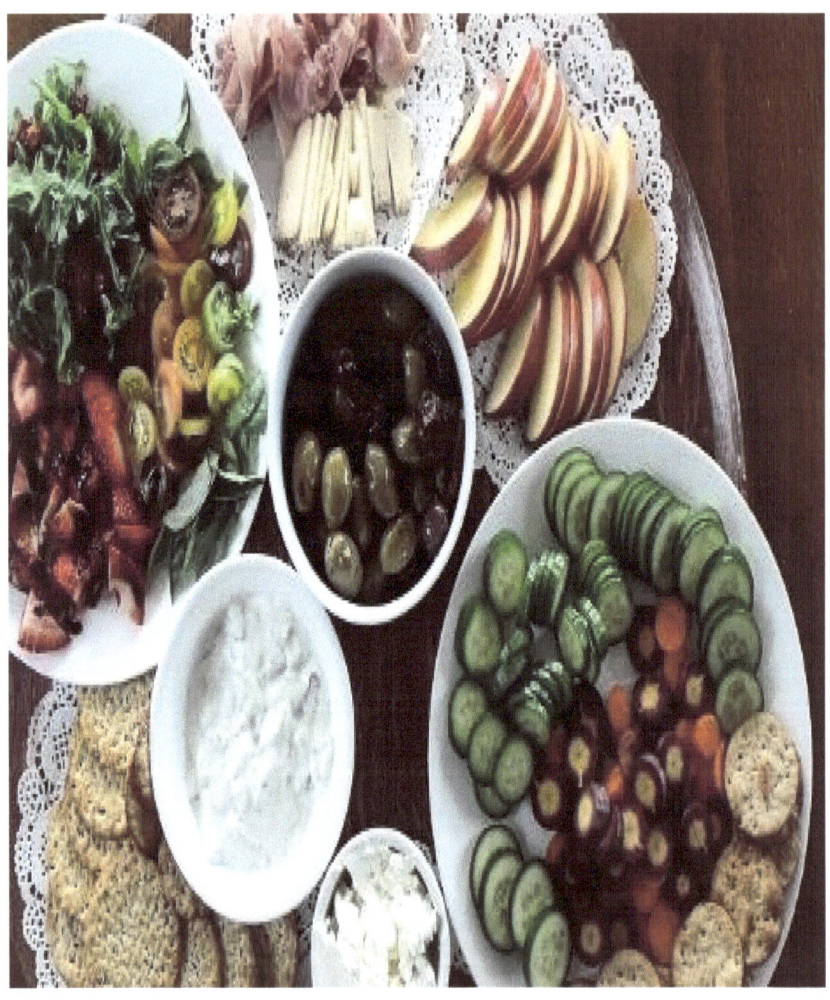

There are countless different exercises and stretches that you can do to work out each of your different ab muscles, but there are a few things that you also must consider that has nothing to do with exercises. I have compiled a list of 4 things to keep in mind if you want to get the most out of your ab exercises.

(1) Make the commitment. You will not achieve your goals if you do not take it seriously. Working your abs hard for 2 days and then slacking off for the remainder of the week will not help you in the long run. If you want to make a change, you must make a commitment to yourself and your routine.

(2) Eat Right. Eating right is critical if you want flatter abs. If you work them really hard and then go home and eat a cheeseburger, all of the good work that you have done has gone out the window. So when you make the commitment, make sure this entails healthy eating.

(3) Do Cardio Exercises. Providing a little variety in your workout is important, and cardio works your abs more than you think.

(4) Do Ab-targeting exercises. It's fine to go to the gym and just do a general workout, but if you really want flat abs, you have to do a lot of exercises that specifically target your abs. If you keep these things in mind, you will be well on your way to flatter abs and a much healthier lifestyle.

Tone Under Arms

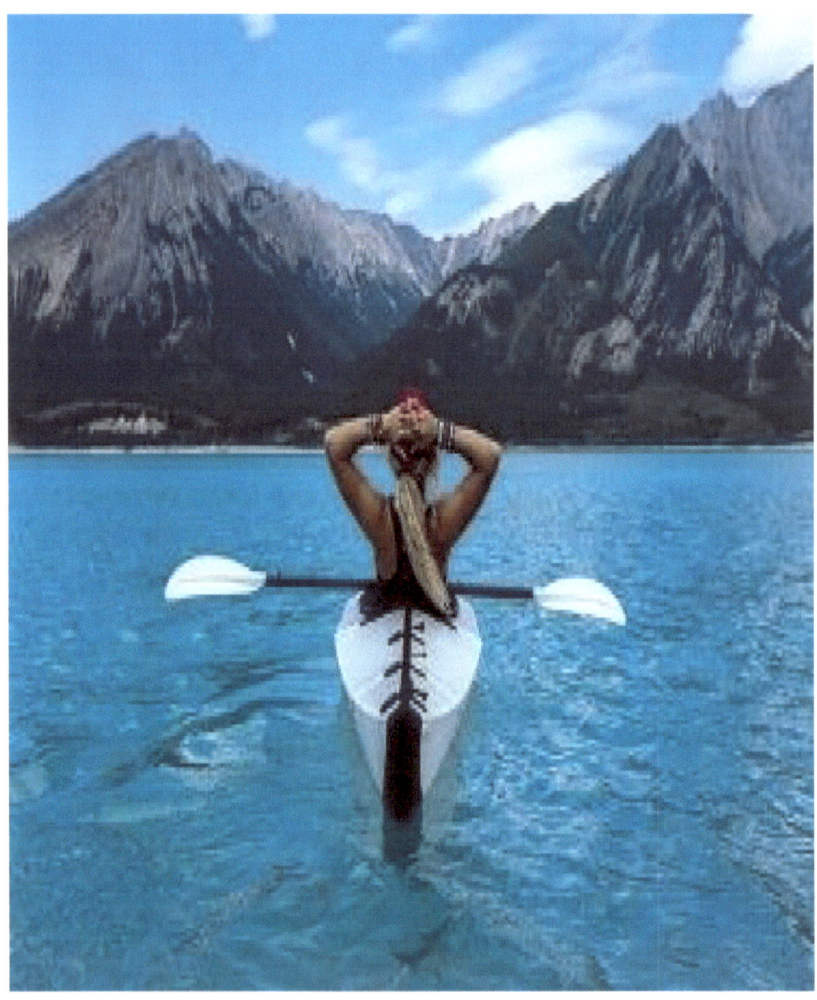

OK, so you want to know how to tone under arms, well then you have stumbled across the right article then. To tone under arms you need to follow a few basic steps. I will discuss some of these steps below and if you are serious about losing weight in your arms and toning them up you should use these tips.

Basic Steps To Follow:

1. You need to rectify your diet to demonstrate healthy eating. The flab you have under your arms is due to fat deposits not burned off throughout the day. Increase your fruit, fibre and vegetable intake.

2. Exercise is a must! It is the only way that you will get rid of the fat around your arms so you can tone them up. Try joining gym, when you see others at the gym with the perfect arms you have always dreamed of, it is bound to motivate you to lose the weight in your arms for good. However as I am sure you already know that not only will you lose weight off your arms, but you will also lose weight of the rest of your body as well.

3. Ensure you do not slack with your cardio exercises. Try running, fast walking and so on, so you can get to your goal quicker by having your heart beat at a fast enough pace to burn of more calories. You should eventually aim for doing this for 20 minutes to a half an hour a day.

4. Push ups are great to tone under arms, it can rely help you firm and define your muscles. This type of exercise uses body weight instead of weights themselves. 5. Using dumb bells between 8 and 10 pounds is also great if you really want to focus on toning your arms while also concentrating on your diet and cardio exercises. Curl you dumb bells as much as you can, aiming to increase the amount each time.

Abdominal Fat: Ways to Reduce It

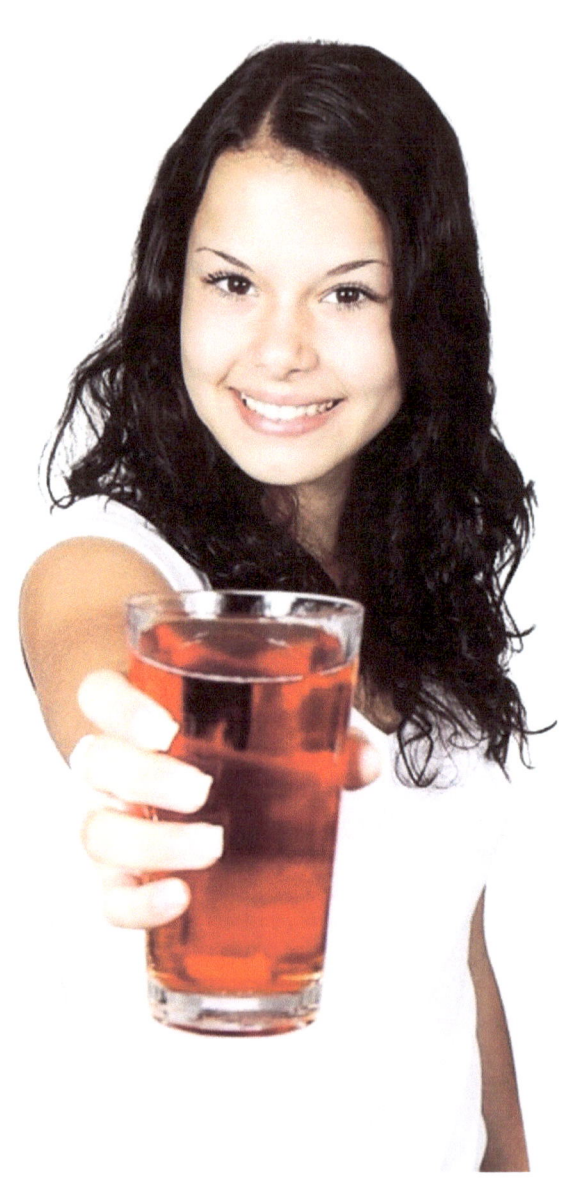

A lean, flat stomach demands time and forbearance for abdominal fat tend to pile up at most tenacious manner in the exercise resistant region. The correct mix of balanced diet, aerobic and cardio exercises, abdominal and weight training can do wonders to burn away abdominal fat and prove more effective than doing sit ups or slaving away with newfangled devices.

The first realization that should dawn on us is that it is impossible to clear away fat from one specific part of body. A majority of people exercise away abdominal areas in vain months after months in the hope that the fat will be burned away directly from that area, but the same only tones and tightens the muscles and the abs remain obscured by abdominal fat. The best means to get rid of layers of flab is cardiovascular exercises.

Aerobic exercises comprising of jogging, bicycling, walking, power stairs etc are the real driving force behind flaccid fat removed. Aerobic exercises must be done for 30-60 minutes each session per day to deplete the glycogen or stored carbohydrate reserves from the body. A fat loss diet comprising of minimal calories must complement the exercises to prevent intake of more calories than being burnt through exercises. The nutritional diet must be spread over into five meals each day to avoid overeating through three regular meals.

Maintain a higher protein and lower carbohydrate rich meal. A major abdominal fat reducing agent is resistance training. Exercising with weights will enhance the lean body mass which subsequently will raise the metabolic rate and quicker the metabolism, the more fat will one burn.

Home Heart Training - 2 Great Cardio Exercises For You to Do at Home!

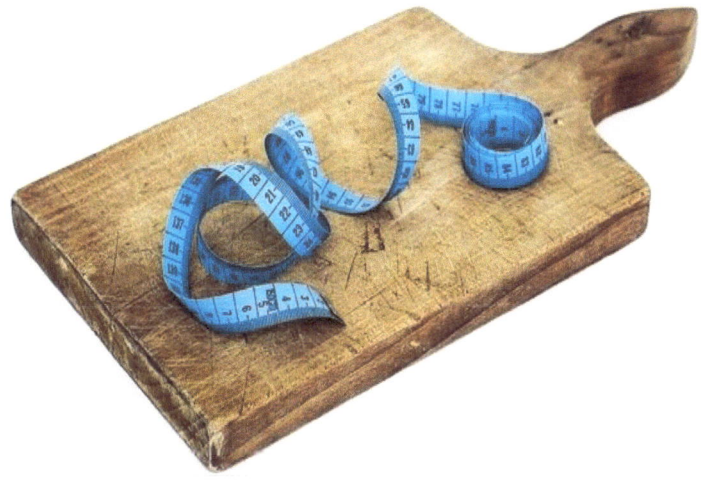

Who says that you can't get a great cardio workout done at home? As a matter of fact, with the right training drills and proper motivation you can get a better cardio workout at home than at a gym in a lot of ways. The best cardiovascular workout has to involve nothing more than your own hand held gym that is known as a kettlebell and a little outdoor yard space. Keep reading if I have your attention. Cardio Conditioning At Home!

1. Kettlebell Snatches To Jump Rope: This is one sick cardio conditioning combination that you can easily perform right in your front yard. With this drill you will simply want to execute a series of kettlebell snatches with a moderately heavy bell with each arm. As soon as you have finished your set of snatches then simply drop the bell on the ground and grab a jump rope and get after it for a duration of 2 minutes. When you have completed the series simply allow yourself a 2 to 3 minute recovery and repeat the process all over again. This is some of the best cardiovascular training you can do anywhere!

2. Kettlebell Totes: For this drill you will need the availability of a couple of bells of moderate resistance and equal weight. From here you are going to utilize the length of your yard to perform some loaded walks with the bells. For this drill the walking surface should be flat, so if your yard isn't a good option then you may want to look into using your driveway, inside hallway, etc. Begin the drill by picking the bells up off of the ground and holding them at your sides. Walk a challenging distance while carrying the bells at your side. You can determine your distance either by measuring or just by simply walking for timed laps. Either way you can make this drill effective by doing so.

Once you begin your loaded walks simply walk the designated distance with the bells at your sides to start. Once you have completed doing this then clean and rack the bells at your chest to perform some loaded walks with them at the rack. This adds additional intensity to the drill and your heart will start really pumping at this point. Once you complete this variation you can take the drill a step further and clean and press the bells overhead to perform the walks. This will add a whole new dynamic of sick strength and unmatched cardio to your workout! If you haven't already started to implement the 2 mentioned cardio drills into your workouts then you are missing out. Take the time to do so and you will have one of the best in home cardio programs going! Remember that most anyone can train hard, but only the best train smart!

Exercise Not Getting Rid of Tummy Fat and Love Handles?

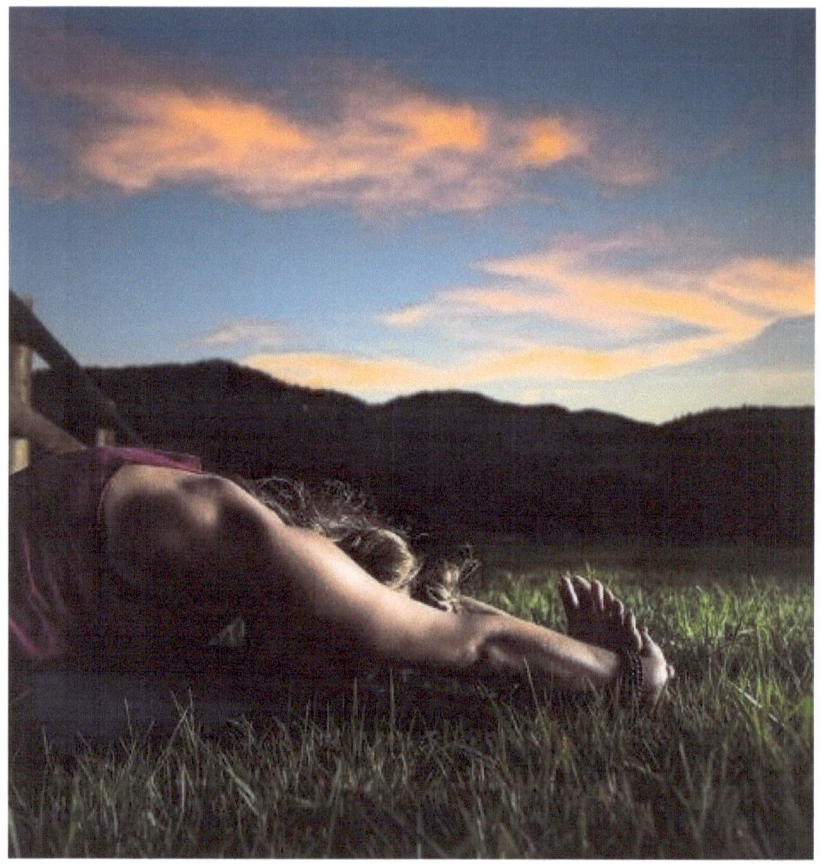

Have you been working out for weeks, months, maybe even years and haven't gotten rid of the weight around your waist? Well, that's because you are probably going about it in the wrong way. But, don't worry because I'm going to tell you exactly what do. But first you need to understand some basics. It takes 3,500 calories of energy to burn a single pound of fat. Now, when you consider that the average person only burns 2,000 calories in an entire 24 hour period then you understand exactly why it is so difficult for people to lose weight.

Most people go about burning fat by doing long cardio exercises such as running or the Stairmaster. However, you can run a few miles and only burn a few hundred calories and still have 3,000 calories to go before you lose your first pound. In the 1990s, however, scientists discovered that if you combine brief periods of exertion with brief periods of rest you can burn more calories and lose more weight in only 4 minutes of exercise a day. So this should be the fundamental format of your exercise routine.

The other thing you should know is that by lifting weights you can burn more fat throughout the day. This is because muscle weighs more than fat and raises your metabolism. Now, if you would like to combine cardio exercises with weight lifting the best way to do this is with a kettlebell. This is a Russian device that, because of its design, enables you to burn as many as 20 calories a minute.

FLAT ABS

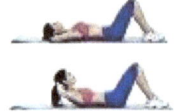
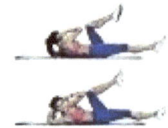
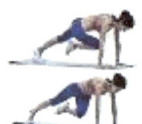

10 CRUNCHES   10 BICYCLE CRUNCHES   10 MOUNTAIN CLIMBERS

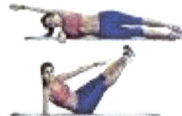
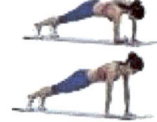
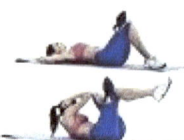

10 SIDE V-UPS (PER SIDE)   10 DYNAMIC PLANKS   10 KNEE TOUCHES

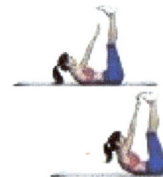
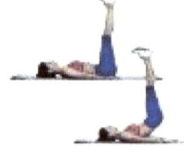
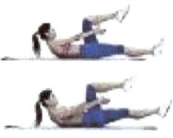

10 TOE TOUCHES   10 LEG LIFTS   10 CRUNCH CLAPS

SETS LEVEL I 2 SETS LEVEL II 3 SETS LEVEL III 4 SETS REST BETWEEN SETS UP TO 1MIN

Your health is your priority. That is the main reason why you want to work out. Working out to look good is the same as working out to be healthy that is why getting a 6 pack abs does not have to be a burden. If you really want to work out, then prioritize your health before aiming to look good. Here are some warnings that you should remember when you are working out on getting a six pack abs. Just like all exercise programs, when you want to get a six pack abs or you just want to tone your stomach, you should still consult your doctor.

As most of the exercises to help you get a six pack abs such as crunches and sit ups may be bad for you especially if you have a lower back problem. So it is always safe to know first before going through these kinds of workouts. Do not forget to do warm-ups. Stretching is always a nice way to start a workout if you do not want to strain your muscles. If you have a few extra pounds, you must know that by doing these exercises, you will look bigger in the midsection as your body builds muscle underneath the fat at first so it is recommended to start on some cardio exercises first before trying to gain a 6 pack abs.

Be careful when eating too much fiber because it also acts like a mild laxative and can cause some gas if you are not used to it. If you increase your fiber dosage, increase your water intake as well. Do not depend on ab machines that you see on TV. It is always best to work out your abs using the floor. A combination of athletic sports, weight lifting, and cardio exercises is a lot more effective for fat loss than an exercise machine. Supplements are just supplements. Meaning they do not have any power to make you lose weight like magic with no work at all. Instead of getting supplements, go for a simple multivitamin or mineral pill as this is what you most likely need.

Sit ups may be bad for your back and neck that is why it should be avoided as much as possible. You can lay on your back and lift your feet in the air as high as you can, and lift your butt off the floor instead. It is a genetic fact that not all women may have the hourglass figure as well as man cannot have the dream chiseled abs. Train your body parts evenly.

Training just one part of your body can be dangerous and might stop you from having the best physique. Drinking too much water is not good too. Too much water in your body might be dangerous as it can dilute certain salts and minerals that are essential to your body. When you need to drink lots of water, supplement it with potassium rich fruits such as bananas or apples.

Using cardio workouts to lose weight can be a highly effective strategy and it can also prove to be a complete waste of time. Mostly, it depends on which workouts you choose to do and how you do them. There's a reason why some people do cardio for years and never seem to lose weight and why others get results quickly. I hope this article will help you do cardio exercises that burn fat and help you get fit. Here are some excellent cardio workouts that you can do to lose fat:

1. Running - My all time favorite workout. You simply can't go wrong with it. If you run regularly and make an effort at it, I'm sure that you're going to see results very quickly. However, to make sure you get the most out of your running activities I recommend that you make sure to run at varying speeds throughout your workout, sometimes slow and sometimes very fast. If you can run at an incline that can also help you to boost your fat loss.

2. Jumping rope - Going outside and working out with a jump rope may seem like a children's game but it can be an effective workout and a very fast one too. Athletes don't do it for no reason. They do it because it just works. It's one of the easiest cardio workouts to do and it's highly effective. Try doing it for 5 minutes and you'll feel how straining it really is. I recommend jumping on a soft surface like grass and not on asphalt or stone as a hard surface can send strong shocks through your body.

3. Aerobic step workouts - To do this right you may need to get a workout DVD or join a class. This will give you more direction in what you're doing. However, I used to get an awesome workout just by switching between one foot and the other with a step. I just place one foot on the step and the other on the floor and then switch between them by jumping, it's an awesome workout to lose weight and can be done at home in front of the TV.

An extra workout you can do is just to take an evening walk. 30 minutes each evening can prove very useful in time. You do need to be aware of the limitation of cardio: unless you also do strength workouts and eat right, you will not get optimal results. However, doing the cardio workouts I wrote about in this article can help you shed pounds fast. That's for sure.

These are some of my other books below, and my website is www.LosingBellyFatMission.com :

https://www.amazon.com/dp/B06XB4WHZX

http://www.amazon.com/dp/B06X9LXBB8

http://www.amazon.com/dp/B06WLK7497

http://www.amazon.com/dp/B06W54JKQN

http://www.amazon.com/dp/B06X6DJ9K3

http://www.amazon.com/dp/B06WGNJ9N3

http://www.amazon.com/dp/B06W549TBD

http://www.amazon.com/dp/B06VTF5DQJ

http://www.amazon.com/dp/B06WRPSBKK

http://www.amazon.com/dp/B06WD194JR

http://www.amazon.com/dp/B06WCZTK7Y

http://www.amazon.com/dp/B06X3QN1HT

http://www.amazon.com/dp/B01N19WBF2

http://www.amazon.com/dp/B01N2AVECA

http://www.amazon.com/dp/B01N4VZIAV

http://www.amazon.com/dp/B00QJJFS1C

http://www.amazon.com/dp/B01EMNO2MW

http://www.amazon.com/dp/B00SSFWCPA

http://www.amazon.com/dp/1520531230

http://www.amazon.com/dp/B01N4V7SR9

http://www.amazon.com/dp/B00SX58DUI

http://www.amazon.com/dp/B010K7YP62

http://www.amazon.com/dp/B012LAYNNQ

http://www.amazon.com/dp/B00RVX3KY2

http://www.amazon.com/dp/B01MR6SWGW

http://www.amazon.com/dp/B00XF6G4HO

http://www.amazon.com/dp/B01F1472N2

http://www.amazon.com/dp/B00PQ0TUPU

http://www.amazon.com/dp/B00PP8OZJ4

http://www.amazon.com/dp/B00QH7DY4Y

http://www.amazon.com/dp/B01052010G
http://www.amazon.com/dp/B00QDHXN7Q
http://www.amazon.com/dp/B00PO0IQIO

Among others.

www.ingramcontent.com/pod-product-compliance
Lightning Source LLC
Chambersburg PA
CBHW050905290526
45792CB00002B/716